EVERYTHING ABOUT THROMBOTIC THROMBOCYTOPENIC PURPURA (TTP)

A Complete Guide For Patients, Caregivers, And Healthcare Professionals - Causes, Symptoms, Diagnosis, Treatment, Coping Strategies + More

DR. CADE JOSUE

Table of Contents

CHAPTER ONE 11
A Synopsis Of Thrombotic Thrombocytopenic Purpura 11
Gaining Insight Into The Pathophysiology Of TTP 12
Symptoms And Clinical Manifestations Of TTP 13
Laboratories And Diagnosis For TTP 15

CHAPTER TWO 19
Methods Of Treatment For TTP 19
Administration Of Acute TTP Episodes 21
Follow-Up And Long-Term Management For TTP Patients 22
Aspects Of Complications Related To TTP: 23
Possible Complications Of TTP Consist Of: .. 23
Outlook And Prognosis For Patients With TTP: 24
Advancements And Research In TTP Treatment 25

CHAPTER THREE 27

   Supportive And Lifestyle Care For TTP Patients
.... 27

   Risk Factors And Epidemiology Of TTP 28

   Trait Variation And Familial TTP 30

   Diagnosis Differential Of TTP 32

CHAPTER FOUR.. 35

   Pregnancy And TTP: Management And
Considerations 35

      Aspects To Consider: 35

      Organizational Management: 36

   Diagnosis And Treatment Of Pediatric TTP In
Children.. 37

      The Diagnosis Is As Follows:........................ 37

      Organizational Management: 38

      Interpersonal Relationship: 39

      Differentiating Factors:................................ 40

   Aspects Of Immunological To TTP 41

      Autoantibodies Consist Of: 41

      Theological Immunology:............................ 42

Treatments Involving Immunomodulatory Agents: 43

CHAPTER FIVE 45

Organ Involvement And TTP: Renal, Neurological, Cardiac, And Additional 45

Clinical Trials And Emerging Therapies For TTP 47

Patient Support And Education Groups For TTP 49

Prospects For The Advancement Of TTP Research And Treatment 50

Summary 53

THE END 55

Copyright © 2024, By Dr. Cade Josue

All Rights Reserved

No part of this book may be reproduced, distributed, or transmitted in any form or by any means, including photocopying, recording, or other electronic or mechanical methods, without the prior written permission of the author, except in the case of brief quotations embodied in Essential reviews and certain other noncommercial uses permitted by copyright law.

DISCLAIMER

The information provided in this book is for general informational purposes only. It is not intended as medical advice, diagnosis, or treatment.

The content of this book should not be considered a substitute for professional medical advice. Readers should consult with a qualified healthcare provider for diagnosis and treatment of any medical conditions they have.

While every effort has been made to ensure the accuracy and completeness of the information presented, the author makes no representations or warranties of any kind, express or implied, about the completeness, accuracy, reliability, suitability, or availability with respect to the information, contained in this book.

The author disclaims any responsibility for any loss or damage resulting from reliance on the information provided in this book. References to individuals, products, websites, organizations, or other names are for informational purposes only and do not imply endorsement.

By reading this book, readers acknowledge that they are responsible for their own health decisions and should seek appropriate medical advice when necessary.

ABOUT THIS BOOK

"Everything About Thrombotic Thrombocytopenic Purpura (TTP)" is an exhaustive book that is considered indispensable reading for medical practitioners, researchers, and individuals in pursuit of a thorough understanding of TTP. This book's structure, which is delineated subsequently, encompasses an extensive array of subjects that are vital for comprehending, diagnosing, treating, and managing TTP.

The introductory section of TTP establishes a fundamental comprehension of the disorder, thereby preparing the reader for a comprehensive examination. Following this, a comprehensive analysis of the pathophysiology of TTP is presented, which illuminates the fundamental mechanisms that propel the progression of the disease. It is critical to comprehend the clinical manifestations and symptoms of TTP to make timely diagnoses and interventions; therefore, the chapter devoted to this subject is a critical component of the book.

Diagnosis and laboratory testing are essential components in the efficient management of TTP. This book explores laboratory methodologies and diagnostic approaches that are crucial for precise diagnosis. Following this, the text delves into treatment methodologies, encompassing both immediate episode management and enduring strategies, thereby providing healthcare practitioners with a comprehensive manual.

In addition, this book discusses patient prognoses, complications associated with TTP, and the most recent developments and research in TTP treatment. By exploring epidemiology, risk factors, and genetic aspects, this work offers a comprehensive analysis of the disorder. The clarification of differential diagnosis, with a specific focus on differentiating TTP from similar conditions, serves to mitigate the risk of misdiagnosis.

Particular considerations such as thrombotic microangiopathy (TMA) and pediatric TTP are extensively examined, in addition to insights into the immunological aspects and association of TTP with TMA. This book also addresses emerging therapies and organ involvement, underscoring the multifaceted nature of TTP management.

Furthermore, this book places significant emphasis on patient education, support groups, and prospective avenues for treatment and research. By adopting a comprehensive approach, healthcare providers are not only informed but also patients and caregivers are equipped with the necessary information and resources to effectively manage TTP.

CHAPTER ONE

A Synopsis Of Thrombotic Thrombocytopenic Purpura

Thrombotic Thrombocytopenic Purpura (TTP) is an uncommon yet critical hematological condition distinguished by thrombosis in minute blood vessels dispersed throughout the organism. Thrombocytopenia is a pathological state characterized by a reduction in the platelet count circulating in the blood and the development of thrombi, which are minute blood clots that affect blood vessels. Blood clots have the potential to obstruct or inhibit the circulation of blood to multiple organs, resulting in harm to tissues and potentially critical complications.

TTP can be broadly categorized into two primary types: congenital TTP and acquired TTP. The incidence of acquired TTP is higher and is predominantly observed in adults, whereas congenital TTP is an early-appearing genetic disorder.

Gaining Insight Into The Pathophysiology Of TTP

A deficiency or dysfunction of the protein ADAMTS13 (a disintegrin and metalloproteinase with a thrombospondin type 1 motif, member 13) is the primary etiological factor associated with TTP. ADAMTS13 is an essential regulator of blood thrombus formation through its cleavage of von Willebrand factor (vWF), a sizable multimeric protein.

A severe deficiency or inhibition of ADAMTS13 activity results in the accumulation of extremely large vWF multimers in the circulation in TTP. Extremely adhesive and capable of spontaneously binding to platelets, these abnormally large vWF multimers facilitate the formation of minute blood clots. The utilization of platelets during the development of these microthrombi further contributes to the condition known as thrombocytopenia.

Ischemia of the tissues and dysfunction of organs result from the extensive development of microthrombi in small blood vessels across the body, with the brain, kidneys, heart, and gastrointestinal tract being particularly affected. Microvascular thrombosis and ischemic injury are fundamental to the pathogenesis of TTP and serve as the foundation for its clinical manifestations.

Symptoms And Clinical Manifestations Of TTP

The clinical manifestation of TTP may differ significantly, yet frequently comprises a pentad of symptoms—although not all patients manifest all five—including:

1. Thrombocytopenia is distinguished by a diminished platelet count in the bloodstream,

which may result in petechiae (minor red or purple discolorations on the skin), mucosal hemorrhage (such as from the pharynx or sinuses), and easy bruising.

2. Microangiopathic hemolytic anemia is caused by the fragmentation of red blood cells as they traverse microthrombi-obstructing tiny blood vessels. Hemoglobinuria (the presence of hemoglobin in the urine) fatigue, pallor, and jaundice (yellowing of the skin and eyes) are potential consequences.

3. Neurological Symptoms: These encompass focal neurological deficits, migraines, confusion, convulsions, and coma; they manifest due to the formation of microthrombi within the cerebral vasculature.

4. Renal dysfunction is characterized by proteinuria, hematuria, decreased urine output,

acute kidney injury resulting from compromised blood flow, and tissue damage within the kidneys.

5. Fever, while infrequent, may manifest in certain patients. This ailment is frequently non-specific in nature and could potentially be attributed to systemic inflammation.

Laboratories And Diagnosis For TTP

The identification of TTP necessitates the integration of imaging studies, laboratory analyses, and clinical assessment. Crucial diagnostic attributes encompass:

1. The complete blood count (CBC) is a diagnostic procedure that commonly detects thrombocytopenia and microangiopathic hemolytic anemia. This is indicated by the presence of schistocytes (fragmented red blood cells), an elevated reticulocyte count, and a low hemoglobin level on peripheral blood smear.

2. A peripheral blood smear analysis may detect schistocytes, which are indicative of microangiopathic hemolytic anemia, a condition that is observed in TTP.

3. Activity Measurement of ADAMTS13: Definitive diagnosis frequently requires activity level measurements of ADAMTS13. ADAMTS13 activity inhibition or a severe deficiency (less than 10% of normal activity) is indicative of TTP.

4. Evaluation of Renal Function: Serum creatinine and blood urea nitrogen (BUN), which are blood tests utilized to assess renal function, might indicate the presence of kidney dysfunction in individuals diagnosed with TTP.

5. Imaging Studies: In patients with neurological symptoms or renal dysfunction, imaging studies such as CT scans or MRIs may be conducted to look for signs of organ injury, particularly in the brain or kidneys.

6. It is critical to rule out alternative etiologies for thrombocytopenia and microangiopathic hemolytic anemia, including disseminated intravascular coagulation (DIC), hemolytic uremic syndrome (HUS), specific infections, and autoimmune disorders.

Treatment must be initiated promptly following a diagnosis to prevent additional organ harm and improve prognoses. Plasma exchange (plasmapheresis) is a common therapeutic approach used to replenish deficient enzyme levels and eliminate circulating inhibitors or antibodies against ADAMTS13.

Additionally, immunosuppressive therapy is employed to impede the immune-mediated elimination of ADAMTS13-producing cells.

Furthermore, as adjunctive therapies, supportive care measures including intravenous fluids, corticosteroids, and blood transfusions may be implemented.

Morbidity and mortality associated with this potentially fatal condition must be drastically reduced through prompt diagnosis and aggressive treatment of TTP.

CHAPTER TWO

Methods Of Treatment For TTP

A combination of therapies designed to reduce platelet aggregation, suppress the immune system (if TTP is autoimmune-mediated), and replace deficient ADAMTS13 enzyme activity are utilized to treat TTP. Principal treatment strategies include:

1. Plasma Exchange (Plasmapheresis): Plasma exchange is the fundamental approach to managing acute TTP. The procedure entails the extraction of the patient's plasma, which comprises pathogenic antibodies and the deficient ADAMTS13 enzyme, and its subsequent substitution with cold-extracted plasma or plasma obtained from healthy donors. By eliminating pathogenic antibodies and reinstating ADAMTS13 activity, this procedure reduces platelet aggregation and improves outcomes.

2. Corticosteroids: In autoimmune-mediated TTP, corticosteroids, such as prednisone, may be combined with plasma exchange to suppress the immune system and decrease the production of pathogenic antibodies.

3. Immunosuppressive Therapy: To target the underlying autoimmune process in cases of autoimmune-mediated TTP or refractory TTP, additional immunosuppressive agents may be administered, such as rituximab (anti-CD20 monoclonal antibody) or cyclophosphamide.

4. ADAMTS13 Replacement Therapy: An emerging treatment approach for TTP is recombinant ADAMTS13 therapy, which entails the administration of exogenous ADAMTS13 enzyme. The objective of this therapeutic approach is to revive impaired ADAMTS13 function and reinstate regular hemostasis.

5. As adjunctive therapies, supportive care may consist of blood transfusions (to rectify anemia and thrombocytopenia), intravenous fluids (to ensure adequate hydration), and symptom-management medications (e.g., pain analgesics).

Administration Of Acute TTP Episodes

Prompt initiation of plasma exchange therapy is essential for the management of acute TTP episodes to eliminate pathogenic antibodies and restore ADAMTS13 activity. Prompt identification and diagnosis are of the utmost importance to avert complications including thromboembolic events and organ injury. It is imperative to closely monitor the platelet count, hemoglobin levels, renal function, and neurological status of patients who are diagnosed with acute TTP. In cases involving organ dysfunction or severe conditions, intensive care support may be required.

Follow-Up And Long-Term Management For TTP Patients

Long-term management of TTP entails continuous monitoring for disease recurrence, evaluation of ADAMTS13 activity levels, and intervention of underlying risk factors, after the resolution of the acute episode.

To avert relapses, patients might necessitate maintenance therapy involving immunosuppressive agents or periodic plasma exchange.

Consistent consultations with hematologists or thrombotic disorders specialists are imperative to maximize long-term results and reduce the occurrence of complications.

Aspects Of Complications Related To TTP:

Possible Complications Of TTP Consist Of:

1. Organ Injury: Prolonged ischemia resulting from microvascular thrombosis has the potential to induce organ injury, with the kidneys, brain, and heart being particularly vulnerable. Risk factors for severe TTP include myocardial infarction, stroke, and renal failure.

2. Thromboembolic Events: TTP elevates the susceptibility to potentially fatal thromboembolic events, including pulmonary embolism (PE), deep vein thrombosis (DVT), and arterial thrombosis, if not administered expeditiously.

3. Neurological complications may arise as a result of TTP, encompassing a spectrum of symptoms that surpass moderate perplexity and headache,

culminating in convulsions, coma, and irreversible neurological deficits.

4. Hematological complications may arise as a result of severe thrombocytopenia and hemolytic anemia. These complications may manifest as hemorrhage, symptoms associated with anemia (e.g., fatigue, lethargy), and compromised coagulation capabilities.

Outlook And Prognosis For Patients With TTP:

Recent years have seen a substantial improvement in the prognosis for TTP due to timely diagnosis and appropriate treatment. As a result of the extensive application of immunosuppressive agents and plasma exchange therapy, the mortality rate has decreased. However, TTP continues to be a condition that poses a risk to life, particularly when not identified and treated promptly.

The severity of the initial presentation, response to treatment, presence of underlying comorbidities, and risk of disease recurrence are all determinants of the prognosis. While there are instances where long-term results may be advantageous, continuous management and vigilant observation are critical for maximizing patient outcomes and quality of life.

Advancements And Research In TTP Treatment

Typically, plasma exchange (also referred to as plasmapheresis) is utilized to treat TTP by removing antibodies and resupplying the deficient ADAMTS13 enzyme. By promptly decreasing circulating antibodies against ADAMTS13 and resupplying the enzyme, plasma exchange effectively inhibits the progression of thrombus formation. In addition, corticosteroids, including prednisone, are frequently employed to inhibit the production of these antibodies by the immune system.

Significant progress has been made in the treatment of TTP in recent years. A noteworthy advancement is the application of caplacizumab, a monoclonal antibody that effectively impedes the interaction between vWF and platelets, thus effectively thwarting the progression of thrombus formation. Caplacizumab has been demonstrated to decrease the recurrence rate of TTP episodes and the time required for platelet count to return to normal.

Moreover, a greater comprehension of the disease mechanisms has resulted from research into the pathogenesis of TTP, which has paved the way for targeted therapies. Ongoing research is examining novel agents that have the potential to increase ADAMTS13 activity or decrease vWF levels; such investigations show promise for enhancing the outcomes of TTP treatment.

CHAPTER THREE

Supportive And Lifestyle Care For TTP Patients

In conjunction with medical intervention, supportive care, and lifestyle adjustments are pivotal components in the management of TTP and the enhancement of patient prognoses. Activities or medications that increase the risk of hemorrhage, such as nonsteroidal anti-inflammatory drugs (NSAIDs) or activities with a high risk of injury, should be avoided by patients with TTP.

Additionally, a balanced diet and regular physical activity are components of a healthy lifestyle that may reduce the risk of complications associated with TTP and enhance overall health. Furthermore, patients undergoing TTP must strictly adhere to their prescribed treatment regimen and consistently attend follow-up consultations with their healthcare providers to assess their condition and make necessary adjustments to their treatment.

TTP patients also require psychological support, given the arduous nature of coping with a chronic and potentially fatal illness. The emotional and psychological aspects of TTP may be better managed by patients and their families through the use of support groups, counseling, and disease education.

Risk Factors And Epidemiology Of TTP

With an estimated annual incidence of 3 to 4 cases per million individuals, TTP is classified as a rare disorder. Although TTP has the potential to manifest at any stage of life, it predominantly impacts adults aged 20 to 50, with a marginal female predilection.

Numerous risk factors have been linked to the onset of TTP, which comprise:

1. Autoimmune disorders: Systemic lupus erythematosus (SLE) and rheumatoid arthritis, in which the immune system attacks the body's tissues, are frequently associated with TTP.

2. Specific infections, especially those caused by viruses like influenza or HIV, have been associated with the emergence of TTP. These infections are thought to induce an immune response that results in the generation of antibodies targeting ADAMTS13.

3. Pharmaceutical Interventions: Several medications, including ticlopidine, clopidogrel, and quinine, have been associated with the occurrence of drug-induced TTP. An immune-mediated response can be induced by these medications, resulting in the generation of antibodies that target ADAMTS13.

4. While uncommon, TTP can manifest during pregnancy or in the immediate postpartum period. Pregnancy-associated TTP is hypothesized to be associated with modifications in hemostatic factors and the immune system.

Trait Variation And Familial TTP

Although TTP is conventionally regarded as an acquired disorder, an increasing body of evidence indicates that certain cases may have a genetic predisposition.

There have been reports of familial cases of TTP, in which several members of the same family are affected, which may indicate the presence of a genetic element in the disease.

In certain patients with familial TTP, mutations in the ADAMTS13 gene, which encodes the ADAMTS13 enzyme, have been identified. These mutations may impair the function or activity of

ADAMTS13, thereby increasing the likelihood of developing TTP.

Furthermore, genetic variations occurring in additional genes that play a role in the regulation of the blood clotting cascade or immune system may potentially contribute to the onset of TTP in specific individuals.

However, additional investigation is required to clarify the precise genetic elements that underlie familial TTP and their function in the development of the disease.

In general, although TTP is predominantly an acquired disorder precipitated by autoimmune or other trigger factors, familial cases suggest that genetic factors may also be significant.

Additional investigation into the genetic underpinnings of TTP could yield valuable knowledge regarding the mechanisms of the disease and possible therapeutic targets.

Diagnosis Differential Of TTP

TTP is differentially diagnosed with several conditions exhibiting comparable clinical manifestations to thrombocytopenia and microangiopathic hemolytic anemia. Possible such conditions comprise:

1. Hemolytic Uremic Syndrome (HUS) is a condition that manifests as acute kidney injury, thrombocytopenia, and microangiopathic hemolytic anemia. An infection with Shiga toxin-producing Escherichia coli (STEC-HUS) or alternative infectious or non-infectious stimuli may elicit this condition.

2. Disseminated intravascular coagulation (DIC) is a consumptive coagulopathy that manifests as a pervasive activation of coagulation pathways,

resulting in platelet and coagulation factor consumption and thrombosis.

It may manifest as a result of a range of underlying conditions, including sepsis, trauma, or cancer.

3. HELLP syndrome, which stands for hemolysis, elevated liver enzymes, and low platelet count, is a profound form of preeclampsia distinguished by thrombocytopenia, elevated liver enzymes, and microangiopathic hemolytic anemia. It manifests predominantly during the course of pregnancy.

4. Drug-induced Thrombotic Microangiopathy (DITMA): Thrombotic microangiopathy approximating TTP can be induced by specific medications, including immunosuppressants, chemotherapeutic agents, and antiplatelet agents. Management requires that the offending agent be discontinued.

5. Atypical Hemolytic Uremic Syndrome (aHUS) is an uncommon hereditary condition distinguished by an imbalance in the complement pathway, which results in thrombotic microangiopathy and endothelial damage. Although it may manifest with comparable clinical symptoms to TTP, complement dysregulation necessitates specialized testing.

CHAPTER FOUR

Pregnancy And TTP: Management And Considerations

TTP during pregnancy presents distinctive difficulties on account of the potential hazards it poses to both the expectant mother and the developing fetus. Pregnancy-associated TTP may manifest in patients with a prior medical history of TTP or previously undiagnosed individuals as a recurrence. A multidisciplinary approach is required for the management of TTP during pregnancy; obstetricians, hematologists, and neonatologists are all involved.

Aspects To Consider:

An elevated risk of TTP is associated with pregnancy as a result of hemostatic alterations and increased levels of vWF.

- Fetal Complications: Untreated uterine thrombocytopenia (TTP) may result in detrimental fetal consequences such as preterm birth, fetal mortality, and intrauterine growth restriction.

- Maternal Complications: TTP presents substantial hazards to the health of the mother, encompassing maternal mortality, renal failure, and stroke.

Organizational Management:

Plasma Exchange (PEX) continues to be the cornerstone of treatment for TTP during pregnancy, to expeditiously eliminate autoantibodies and restore ADAMTS13 activity.

- Vigilant Monitoring: Pregnant women diagnosed with TTP must undergo regular evaluations of fetal and maternal health, such as platelet count, renal function, and fetal growth.

- Delivery Timing: Maternal and fetal factors, including the severity of transplacement fetal preterm birth (TTP) and gestational age, should inform the determination of the optimal timing of delivery.

Diagnosis And Treatment Of Pediatric TTP In Children

TTP in children is an uncommon yet critical condition that demands immediate identification and intervention. Even though the clinical manifestation of TTP in children is comparable to that of adults, pediatric patients present with distinct challenges when it comes to diagnosis and treatment.

The Diagnosis Is As Follows:

- Clinical Presentation: In addition to lethargy, pallor, and petechiae, children with TTP may exhibit neurologic abnormalities and renal dysfunction, among other severe manifestations.

• Laboratory Results: The presence of thrombocytopenia, microangiopathic hemolytic anemia, and end-organ injury are indicative of the diagnosis. Activity testing for ADAMTS13 could potentially aid in the validation of the diagnosis.

Organizational Management:

Plasma Exchange (PEX) is the primary therapeutic approach for pediatric TTP, mirroring its use in adults. Its objective is to eliminate autoantibodies and restore ADAMTS13 activity.

• Pediatric Considerations: Weight, vascular access, and the necessity for analgesia or anesthesia during PEX are some of the variables that may necessitate modifications to treatment in pediatric patients.

• Multidisciplinary Care: A multidisciplinary team comprising pediatric hematologists, intensivists, and pediatric nurses with expertise in the management of critically ill children may be necessary to provide care for pediatric patients with TTP.

Differentiating TTP from Thrombotic Microangiopathy (TMA) and Their Interrelation

TTP is a subtype of thrombotic microangiopathy (TMA), an assemblage of conditions distinguished by dysfunction of the organs and microvascular thrombosis. Although TTP is a clearly defined condition, its relationship to other TMAs, including Hemolytic Uremic Syndrome (HUS) and Atypical Hemolytic Uremic Syndrome (aHUS), must be acknowledged.

Interpersonal Relationship:

• Pathophysiological Similarities: Microangiopathic hemolytic anemia, thrombocytopenia, and microvascular thrombosis are shared characteristics among TTP, HUS, and aHUS. Nevertheless, the fundamental mechanisms vary.

• ADAMTS13 Deficiency: TTP is distinguished by a profound insufficiency of ADAMTS13 activity, which results in the formation of platelet-rich microthrombi and the accumulation of ultra-large vWF multimers.

• Complement Dysregulation: aHUS is characterized by endothelial injury and thrombotic microangiopathy due to dysregulation of the complement pathway.

Differentiating Factors:

• Underlying Mechanisms: Although ADAMTS13 deficiency is the primary cause of TTP, infection with Shiga toxin-producing bacteria (STEC-HUS), complement dysregulation (aHUS), or other stimuli may lead to HUS.

• Clinical Characteristics: TTP frequently manifests with a pentad of symptoms, comprising renal dysfunction, neurologic abnormalities, and fever, whereas HUS may manifest with acute kidney injury and gastrointestinal symptoms.

• Treatment: Plasma exchange (PEX) is utilized to eliminate autoantibodies and restore ADAMTS13 activity in the management of TTP. Conversely, supportive care and, in certain instances, antibiotics or eculizumab for aHUS may be prescribed for the treatment of HUS.

Aspects Of Immunological To TTP

Significant immunological aspects are associated with thrombotic thrombocytopenic purpura (TTP), most notably the formation of autoantibodies that target ADAMTS13 and the resultant disruption of von Willebrand factor (vWF) metabolism's normal regulation.

Autoantibodies Consist Of:

• Anti-ADAMTS13 Antibodies: Acquired TTP is characterized by the development of autoantibodies against ADAMTS13 in the patient, which impairs vWF cleavage and decreases enzyme activity.

• IgG Subtype: The IgG subtype comprises the preponderance of anti-ADAMTS13 antibodies. These antibodies bind to ADAMTS13 and impede its activity, thereby facilitating the accumulation of ultra-large vWF multimers.

Theological Immunology:

• B-cell Activation: The generation of autoantibodies against ADAMTS13 is facilitated through the activation of B cells, which is required for the production of anti-ADAMTS13 antibodies.

• T-cell Participation: T cells potentially contribute to the development of TTP through their facilitation of B-cell activation and generation of antibodies targeting ADAMTS13.

• Genetic Predisposition: Although acquired TTP is predominantly linked to autoantibodies, susceptibility to developing anti-ADAMTS13 antibodies may be influenced by underlying genetic predispositions.

Treatments Involving Immunomodulatory Agents:

• Corticosteroids: Corticosteroids are frequently employed as supplementary therapies in TTP to modulate the immune response and inhibit autoantibody production.

Rituximab, a monoclonal antibody targeting CD20, has demonstrated efficacy in decreasing levels of anti-ADAMTS13 antibodies and promoting remission in patients with refractory or relapsing tumor proliferative disease (TTP).

• Potential Future Directions: Further investigation into innovative immunomodulatory therapies, including proteasome inhibitors or B-cell targeting compounds, could provide supplementary therapeutic alternatives for TTP.

Gaining insight into the immunological dimensions of TTP is of the utmost importance to advance the design of targeted treatments that seek to regulate the immune response and reinstate regular ADAMTS13 operation. Such advancements would ultimately benefit patients afflicted with this uncommon and potentially fatal condition.

CHAPTER FIVE

Organ Involvement And TTP: Renal, Neurological, Cardiac, And Additional

A rare yet severe blood disorder, TTP is distinguished by the development of thromboses in minute blood vessels across the entirety of the organism. Various organs may be harmed by these blockages, which may result in severe complications.

• Renal Involvement: TTP frequently impacts the kidneys. Renal failure can occur as a result of clot formation in the small blood vessels of the kidneys; symptoms include reduced urinary output, inflammation, and electrolyte imbalances.

• Neurological Involvement: Clot formation in the cerebral artery arteries frequently results in neurological symptoms in TTP patients. This may lead to a spectrum of symptoms, including but not limited to moderate confusion, migraines, seizures, strokes, and coma.

• Cardiac Involvement: While infrequent, TTP has the potential to impact the heart through the formation of thrombi in the blood vessels that supply the myocardium. This may result in symptoms including dyspnea, chest discomfort, and, in critical instances, myocardial infarction.

• Involvement of Other Organs: TTP has the potential to impact various other organs, including the epidermis, gastrointestinal tract, and lungs. Symptoms that may result from clot formation in these organs include respiratory difficulties, abdominal pain, vertigo, vomiting, and purpura (fine purple or red patches on the skin).

Clinical Trials And Emerging Therapies For TTP

In light of recent progress in comprehending the pathogenesis of TTP, targeted therapies have been created to impede the development of blood clotting and enhance patient prognoses. The following are examples of ongoing clinical trials and emerging therapies for TTP:

• ADAMTS13 Replacement Therapy: TTP is characterized by a deficiency or dysfunction of the von Willebrand factor-cleaving enzyme ADAMTS13. As a prospective treatment option, replacement therapy with recombinant ADAMTS13 or plasma-derived ADAMTS13 concentrates is being investigated.

Monoclonal antibodies, which selectively target particular components of the coagulation cascade (e.g., platelet glycoprotein Ib or von Willebrand factor (VWF)), are currently under investigation to impede the development of atypical blood clots in TTP.

• Novel Antiplatelet Agents: The effectiveness of novel antiplatelet agents with distinct mechanisms of action in preventing platelet aggregation and thrombus formation in TTP is currently being assessed.

• Gene Therapy: As prospective long-term interventions for TTP, gene therapy strategies that correct the underlying genetic defects responsible for ADAMTS13 deficiency or dysfunction are being investigated.

To evaluate the safety and efficacy of these emerging therapies and to further our understanding of the pathophysiology of TTP, clinical trials are indispensable.

Patient Support And Education Groups For TTP

As a result of the rarity and severity of TTP, patient support and education are vital for enhancing prognoses and quality of life. Patient education ought to center on:

• Disease Understanding: Delivering extensive information to patients and their families regarding TTP, encompassing its etiology, manifestations, diagnostic criteria, therapeutic alternatives, and possible adverse effects.

• Medication Management: Disseminating knowledge to patients regarding the significance of adhering to prescribed medications, potential adverse effects associated with treatment, and effective symptom management and disease flare-up prevention strategies.

Encourage patients to embrace lifestyle modifications that promote well-being, such as engaging in consistent physical activity, adhering to a well-balanced diet, ceasing tobacco use, and avoiding stimuli that could intensify symptoms of TTP.

• Emotional Support: Provide counseling and emotional support to assist patients in managing the psychological effects associated with having a chronic and potentially fatal condition.

Peer support, practical guidance, and the exchange of personal experiences are all valuable contributions that support groups for TTP patients and their families can offer. Healthcare professionals, patient advocacy organizations, or virtual communities may facilitate these groups.

Prospects For The Advancement Of TTP Research And Treatment

Subsequent lines of inquiry in TTP seek to enhance our understanding of the fundamental mechanisms at play within the disorder while also devising targeted and individualized therapeutic approaches. Potential areas of concentration may encompass:

• Biomarker Discovery: The identification of previously unidentified biomarkers that are linked to the pathogenesis and progression of TTP to facilitate early diagnosis, risk stratification, and treatment response monitoring.

• Precision Medicine: The application of genomic and proteomic methodologies to discern molecular profiles and genetic variations specific to individual patients that could potentially impact the susceptibility, severity, and therapeutic response to TTP.

• Immunomodulatory Therapies: Examining the involvement of the immune system in the pathophysiology of TTP and investigating innovative immunomodulatory treatments to manage the condition, including immune checkpoint inhibitors and cytokine-targeted therapies.

• Regenerative Medicine: Investigating the potential of regenerative medicine methodologies, including tissue engineering and stem cell therapy, to restore and regenerate impaired blood vessels and organs in patients with TTP.

• Patient-Centered Outcomes Research: Undertaking patient-centered outcomes research to assess the influence of TTP on the quality of life, functional status, and psychosocial well-being of patients. Additionally, this research aims to identify any unresolved issues and establish priorities for future clinical care and research.

By addressing these research priorities and fostering collaboration among multidisciplinary teams, we can develop more effective strategies for the prevention, diagnosis, and treatment of TTP and increase our understanding of the disease.

Summary

In summary, Thrombotic Thrombocytopenic Purpura (TTP) is an uncommon yet critical medical condition distinguished by the development of thromboses in minute blood vessels across the entirety of the organism.

TTP is frequently caused by an enzyme deficiency in ADAMTS13, which is critical for the enzymatic degradation of von Willebrand factor (vWF), a protein that is integral to the process of blood clotting.

Prompt diagnosis and immediate treatment initiation are essential components in the effective management of TTP to avert severe complications, including organ damage and mortality. Plasma exchange therapy continues to be the fundamental approach in managing acute TTP episodes, as it seeks to substitute the deficient ADAMTS13 enzyme. Furthermore, to mitigate the atypical immune response, corticosteroids or rituximab, which are immunosuppressive drugs, may be administered.

A greater comprehension of the pathogenesis of TTP and the development of novel therapies, such as caplacizumab, a monoclonal antibody that inhibits platelet aggregation and targets vWF, are the results of advances in medical research. Notwithstanding these therapeutic progressions, TTP remains a formidable obstacle on account of its capricious characteristics and relapse propensity.

Comprehensive management of TTP requires a multidisciplinary approach encompassing hematologists, nephrologists, and other specialists. This approach should prioritize early detection, aggressive treatment, and long-term monitoring to enhance patient outcomes and quality of life.

THE END